MW01644309

Table of Contents

Introduction

Cannabis in skin care may be seen as a marijuana advertising technique, yet the plant is full of fixings that are valuable in more than simply a joint. Hemp hails from eastern Asia and it can be followed back thousands of years to ancient India and China, where it was used in medicine as an hostile to maturing item. It was also used to stimulate and enhance blood dissemination. Both hemp and cannabis come from different parts of the cannabis sativa plant.

Despite its association with cannabis, hemp is free of tetrahydrocannabinol (THC), which is the stimulating associated with marijuana.scientists are uncovering many uses for marijuana, and there's a growing body of research revealing its impacts on our skin. Studies propose that poisonous side-effects from marijuana smoke may increase skin aging. Yet, other exploration shows that beneficial compounds in marijuana may improve the skin. Those who are concerned about showing their age should stay away from smoking maryjane and grasp edibles, vaporizing, and pot based topicals instead.Many changes in the body lead to aging of the skin. After the age of 20, the skin produces 1% less collagen each year. Collagen helps the skin show up firm and supple, and losing it makes the skin thinner and more fragile. Likewise, your skin produces less oil as you age, making it drier. This is why saturating gets more and more important as we age. Sun exposure can likewise cause damage to the skin which contributes to aging and skin malignant growth. Finally, environmental toxins contribute to the aging process. This is why people who smoke cigarettes regularly look older than non-smokers of the same age.

Marijuana contains incredible enemy of inflammatories and antioxidants which can ensure the skin against harm caused by natural openness. An examination published by the National Academy of Sciences in 1998 found that the cannabinoid CBD is an all the more impressive cell reinforcement than Vitamins E and

C. THC was also discovered to have antioxidant properties. Cell reinforcements protect the skin by killing free extremists. Free radicals are unstable molecules that harm the cells in your body and cause all sorts of damage, from aging to malignancy. The amazing antioxidants in marijuana may battle maturing by ensuring the cells in your body against free radical damage. Marijuana items have likewise been reported to help treat more serious skin problems, such as malignant growth. Marijuana activist Rick

Simpson broadly used cannabis imbued oil to heal a cancerous growth on his arm. He was already using marijuana oil therapeutically, so he tried applying some on the development straightforwardly. Simpson checked his skin after a few days. To his surprise, the carcinoma was gone. Simpson believes the cannabis oil treated his skin cancer where traditional methods failed. Marijuana's effects on skin cancer show up to be more than just anecdotal. A 2003 study found that treatment with cannabinoids caused skin cancer cells to bite the dust, while leaving healthy cells safe. The trial was repeated in living mice with skin tumors and the same results were found. Human preliminaries have not been done yet, however the proof so far is promising. Cannabis imbued skin creams can also be used to treat rashes, dry skin, and more genuine skin conditions like dermatitis and psoriasis thanks to their anti-inflammatory properties.

what is cannabis

Cannabis in skin care may be seen as a marijuana showcasing technique, yet the plant is full of fixings that are helpful in more than simply a joint. Hemp hails from eastern Asia and it can be followed back thousands of years to ancient India and China, where it was used in medicine as an hostile to maturing item. It was also used to stimulate and enhance blood flow. Both hemp and cannabis come from different parts of the cannabis sativa plant.

Despite its association with cannabis, hemp is free of tetrahydrocannabinol (THC), which is the psychedelic associated with marijuana.scientists are uncovering many uses for marijuana, and there's a growing body of research revealing its impacts on our skin. Studies recommend that harmful results from marijuana smoke may increase skin aging. Yet, other examination shows that beneficial compounds in marijuana may improve the skin. Those who are concerned about showing their age should stay away from smoking weed and grasp edibles, vaporizing, and maryjane based topicals instead.Many changes in the body lead to aging of the skin. After the age of 20, the skin produces 1% less collagen each year. Collagen helps the skin show up firm and supple, and losing it makes the skin thinner and more weak. Additionally, your skin produces less oil as you age, making it drier. This is why saturating gets more and more important as we age. Sun exposure can likewise cause damage to the skin which contributes to aging and skin disease. Finally, environmental contaminations contribute to the aging process. This is why people who smoke cigarettes frequently look older than non-smokers of the same age. Marijuana contains incredible enemy of inflammatories and antioxidants which can secure the skin against harm caused by ecological openness. An examination published by the National Academy of Sciences in 1998 found that the cannabinoid CBD is an all the more remarkable cell reinforcement than Vitamins E and C. THC was also discovered to have antioxidant properties. Cell reinforcements protect the skin by killing free revolutionaries. Free radicals are unstable molecules that harm the cells in your body and cause all sorts of damage, from aging to malignant growth. The incredible antioxidants in marijuana may battle maturing by securing the cells in your body against free radical damage. Marijuana items have likewise been reported to help treat more serious skin problems, such as disease. Marijuana activist Rick Simpson broadly used maryjane mixed oil to heal a cancerous growth on his arm. He was already using marijuana oil restoratively, so he tried applying some on the development straightforwardly. Simpson checked his skin after a few days. To his surprise, the carcinoma was gone. Simpson believes the cannabis oil treated his skin cancer where traditional methods failed. Marijuana's effects on skin cancer show up to be more than just anecdotal. A 2003 study found that treatment with cannabinoids caused skin cancer cells to pass on, while leaving healthy cells safe. The examination was repeated in living mice with skin tumors and the same results were found. Human preliminaries have not been done yet, yet the proof so far is promising. Maryjane mixed skin creams can also be used to treat rashes, dry skin, and more genuine skin conditions like dermatitis and psoriasis thanks to their anti-inflammatory properties.

Types of Cannabis and Health Risks

With states authorizing across the country, numerous individuals are beginning to learn that there are various varieties of the cannabis plant, sometimes called "weed", and they can be arranged in a variety of ways. The potency of cannabis can vary greatly from one plant to another and from one preparation to another. The route of administration can strongly influence the power of marijuana's impacts. One individual's experience of taking marijuana can be completely diverse from that of someone else.

Smoking Weed

Regularly simply called weed or pot, this is the unprocessed form of cannabis. Weed consists of the dried leaves and buds of the female Cannabis sativa and Cannabis indica plants. It has a very pungent and conspicuous odor, both in its unburnt state and while being smoked. This smell is very dissimilar to kitchen herbs, despite the fact that weed is now and then "cut" (mixed) with favorable kitchen herbs such as oregano and parsley when sold in the underground market. Weed is commonly smoked in hand-moved cigarettes, known as joints. The uneven texture of weed can be felt through the tobacco moving paper. This is one of the characteristics that can differentiate a joint from a hand-rolled tobacco cigarette. Hashish and weed can be blended with rolling tobacco, which is a soft, moist, sticky tobacco planning designed for hand-rolling. It may also be mixed with the dry tobacco from deconstructed cigarettes. This mixture is alluded to as a "spliff". Weed, hashish, and hashish oil can be smoked in pipes, water pipes, and bongs, or blended in with tobacco and smoked in a chillum. Some youthful adults have also used e-cigarettes to inhale marijuana through "vaping.

Hashish

Hashish, or hash for short, is a readiness of marijuana made from the tar of the Cannabis sativa or Cannabis indica plant. The resin is dried into blocks of hashish, producing an oily, solid substance. Cannabis resin can be alluded to by the names for the particular type of hash, rather than the generic names of hashish or pot. These diverse names for hashish include black, goldseal black, redseal black, and Morrocan (Rocky for short). Hashish is regularly warmed, crumbled, and moved together with tobacco. It might also be smoked in a line, bong, or chillum. There are several different types of hashish. The colors range from dark brown or nearly black, through various shades of earthy colored, to a dirty yellowish color. The appearance of changed sorts of hashish can vary as well. Some may look dark and shiny (a bit like licorice) and some may be lighter and dull or matte (a bit like a soup stock block). The surface of hashish also varies from very dry and hard, like a piece of fudge, to moist and flexible, like demonstrating clay. As with weed, hashish has a very distinctive, impactful odor. It is one of the most straightforward ways of distinguishing it as a structure of maryjane. The appearance of hashish is so changed that beginner users are often tricked into purchasing licorice or other cheap, benign substances that look similar. Hashish oil, or hash oil, is the strongest form of marijuana and is the least common type of the drug.It is sold in tiny bottles or fixed plastic packs. Only a small sum is required to produce the effects of weed. Typically, hash oil is smoked in a line or painted onto cigarettes or joints.

Cannabis-Infused Food and Drink

Marijuana can likewise be taken orally and is often prepared into food. In this form, it is commonly called edibles. An exemplary way to eat marijuana is in the structure of brownies or cookies. However, maryjane can be added to many types of food, just like an spice, and may even appear in candy.

Hashish and hashish oil can be dissolved into milk and consumed in drinks. Milk is the transporter of decision due to its emulsive properties as cannabis is an oil-based substance. With palatable forms of maryjane, it takes longer to feel the psychoactive effects and it can be quite potent.

what are the components of cannabis?

Cannabis is made up of more than 120 components, which are known as cannabinoids. Experts still aren't sure what each cannabinoid does, yet they have a pretty good understanding of two of them, known as cannabidiol (CBD) and tetrahydrocannabinol (THC).

Each has its own impacts and employments:

CBD. This is a psychoactive cannabinoid, yet it's non-intoxicating and non-euphoric, meaning it won't get you "high." It's often used to help lessen irritation and pain. It may also ease nausea, migraine, seizures, and anxiety. (Epidiolex is the first and only prescription medication to contain CBD and be approved by the Food and Drug Administration, or FDA. This medication is used to treat specific sorts of epilepsy.) Researchers are still attempting to completely comprehend the effectiveness of CBD's medical use. THC. This is the principle psychoactive compound in cannabis. THC is mindful for the "high" that most individuals partner with cannabis.

Health Benefits of Cannabis

Relief of chronic pain

There are hundreds of synthetic compounds in cannabis, numerous of which are cannabinoids. Cannabinoids have been connected to providing relief of persistent agony due to their chemical cosmetics. Which is why cannabis' by-product, for example, clinical cannabis is commonly used for chronic torment relief.

Improves lung capacity

Unlike smoking cigarettes, when smoking cannabis in the structure of cannabis your lungs aren't harmed. In fact, a study found that cannabis actually helps increment the limit of the lungs rather than cause any mischief to it.

Help get in shape

On the off chance that you look around, you will notice that the avid cannabis user is usually not overweight. That is on the grounds that cannabis is connected to helping your body in regulating insulin while managing caloric intake efficiently.

Regulate and prevent diabetes

With its effect on insulin, it just makes sense that cannabis can help manage and prevent diabetes. Examination conducted by the American Alliance for Medical Cannabis (AAMC) has linked cannabis to stabilise blood sugars, lower blood pressure, and improve blood circulation.

Fight malignant growth

One of the greatest medical benefits of cannabis is its connection to battling cancer. There is a decent amount of evidence that shows cannabinoids can help fight cancer or at least certain types of it.

Helps treat depression

Discouragement is fairly widespread without most people even knowing they have it. The endocannabinoid compounds in cannabis can help in stabilising mind-sets which can ease depression.

Shows guarantee in chemical imbalance treatment

Cannabis is known to quiet users down and control their mood. It can help children with chemical imbalance that experience successive violent state of mind swings control it.

Regulate seizures

Research led on CBD has shown that it can help control seizures. There are ongoing considers to decide the impact cannabis has on people with epilepsy.

Mend bones

Cannabidiol has been connected to helping heal broken bones, quickening the measure. According to Bone Research Laboratory in Tel Aviv, it additionally helps strengthen the bone in the process of recuperating. This makes it tougher for the bone to break in what's to come.

Helps with ADHD/ADD

Individuals with ADHD and ADD have inconvenience focusing on tasks at hand. They tend to have issues with cognitive execution and focus. Cannabis has shown guarantee in promoting center and aiding individuals with ADHD/ADD. It is also considered a safer alternative to Adderall and Ritalin.

Treatment for glaucoma

Glaucoma leads to additional pressure on the eyeball which is difficult for individuals with the disorder. Cannabis can help reduce the pressure applied on the eyeball giving some temporary relief to people with glaucoma.

Lighten anxiety

While Cannabis is commonly known to cause anxiety, there is a way around that. Taken in checked measurement and in the appropriate way, cannabis can help alleviate anxiety and calm clients down.

Slow development of Alzheimer's illness

Alzheimer's disease is one of many that is caused by cognitive degeneration. As we age, cognitive degeneration is almost unavoidable. Cannabis's endocannabinoid contains hostile to inflammatories that fight the brain irritation that leads to Alzheimer's disease.

Arrangement with pain linked to joint inflammation

Cannabis is now usually found as creams and balms which are used by individuals that have joint pain. Both THC and CBD help sufferers bargain with the agony.

Helps with PTSD symptoms

PTSD doesn't simply affect veterans however any individual that goes through a trauma. As cannabis is legalised the impact it has on helping treat individuals with PTSD is being studied. Cannabis helps control the fight or flight reaction, forestalling it from going into overdrive.

Encourages provide help to individuals with multiple sclerosis

Multiple sclerosis can be painful, and cannabis is known to give help for it. Multiple sclerosis leads to agonizing muscle contractions and cannabis can help reduce that pain.

Reduces side effects linked to hepatitis C and increment the effectiveness of treatment

The treatment for hepatitis C has numerous side effects that incorporate sickness, weakness, depression, and muscle aches.

These can last for months for some hepatitis C sufferers. Cannabis can help reduce the results caused by the treatment while making it more powerful at the same time.

Treats inflammatory bowel illnesses

Individuals with Crohn's illness or ulcerative colitis can find some relief with the use of cannabis. THC and cannabidiol are known to help enhance immune response while also interact with cells that play an essential role in the working of the gut. Cannabis helps close off bacteria and different mixes that cause inflammation in the digestive organs.

Helps with quakes associated with Parkinson's disease

For those that have Parkinson's disease cannabis can help diminish quakes and pain while also helping promote rest. It has also shown to improve motor skills in patients.

Helps with alcoholism

Another of the many wellbeing benefits of cannabis is that there is no doubt cannabis is a lot more secure than liquor. While it may not be 100% risk-free, it can be a more intelligent way to curb liquor abuse by substituting it with cannabis.

Hemp in skin health management cannabis

Our skin protects us against viruses, bacteria and abundance water loss. Collagen gives solidness and elasticity for our skin. After the age of 20, our skin production of collagen drops 1% per year and this leads to the skin appearing thinner and more brittle. Maturing also comes with drier skin and the measure is quickened due to sun exposure. Through all things considered, our skin can sometimes fail to do its job and so skin care products come into play. Scientists are uncovering numerous uses for weed, and there's a growing body of research uncovering its effects on our skin. The notion of marijuana in skincare may seem like another argument to legalize the medication yet this is not the situation. Hemp has been a fixture in skin care products for various years. Besides, pesticides and herbicides are not utilized in the cultivating of hemp seed so there is no dread of pesticide buildup in your skin care items. A 1998 National Academy of Sciences study claimed that hemp is a more powerful cell reinforcement when compared to

Vitamins E and C. The cancer prevention agents kill free extremists precarious molecules that can cause aging as well as skin cancer. The balance of Omega-6 and Omega-3 unsaturated fats found in hemp seeds is seen as the ideal element for healthy cell production and good skin health. Hemp seeds can also produce hemp oil and this multipurpose oil is full of essential nutrients. The oil can be used for hair care-advancing hair growth and preventing hair loss. The oil can also relieve irritation and dryness as well as forestall dandruff from shaping. As it improves blood flow and reduces aggravation, the oil will help keep scalp diseases away. Hemp seed oil is great for your beauty system as it is non-comedogenic and it penetrates the skin easily. The oil assists with moisture misfortune, untimely aging and it likewise lightens skin conditions like dermatitis, acne and psoriasis. According to a Journal of Dermatological Treatment study, hemp seed helped to alleviate side effects of dermatitis after 20 weeks.

Hemp in our weight control plans

Hemp oil can be used to cook and plan food. It is low in immersed fat and this makes it a superior option than butter.cannabis | Longevity LIVEIt also contains sitosterol which can help lower cholesterol and this thus reduces the danger of heart disease.The antioxidant properties found in the oil can help prevent your cell damage and are also anti-cancer agents. The oil also contains vitamins and minerals going from calcium and potassium to Vitamins B-6 and E. A

2007 study viewed hemp as a viable protein alternative for individuals who avoid animal products. The protein can be processed and utilized more effectively due to the concentration of its amino acids. The protein absorbability of the seed was more than, and equivalent to other protein sources such as grains and nuts. As beneficial as hemp seeds are, they are also high in calories with 170 calories for every 3-tablespoon serving. It is recommended that you use them in small portions and ideally use them as your sole protein source.

Does hemp make smoking cannabis a better option

The smoke from cannabis can be detrimental to the skin, speeding up the aging process. Furthermore, it produces toxic results – to be specific free radicals and cancer-causing agents. The smoke can likewise meddle with collagen production and this can lead to dry and brittle skin. On the off chance that you suffer from psoriasis, smoking maryjane can worse the condition. Smoking marijuana can likewise affect your testosterone levels, which impacts sebum creation.

How To Use Marijuana For Healthy Skin

The method of utilization is important when using marijuana to improve and protect your skin. Disintegrating has gained in popularity in ongoing years. Vaporizers heat marijuana to the point where its beneficial cannabinoids are delivered in a gas that can be inhaled. This avoids creating the harmful toxins found in smoke. Edibles are another smokeless method of consuming cannabis and its health-promoting fixings. Cannabis edibles are foods that have been injected with cannabis. Like disintegrating, edibles allow you to consume marijuana's beneficial compounds while avoiding exposure to any harmful or harming side-effects. The best way to use marijuana to improve your skin is to use an injected topical product. On the off chance that you have access to a dispensary, they will likely have a determination of cannabis based creams and oils made by licensed manufacturers.

Benefit of Cannabis to the skin

Of the numerous organs of the human body, there is none larger than skin. It literally wraps our entire organism, and it works in ways that are characteristic of the overall state of the body. On the off chance that there's a medical issue going on inside us, there is a good chance that our skin will manifest some symptoms. For example, skin dehydration is one of the most common sicknesses that affect this organ. It can often be set off by congestion or other regular medical problems. However, there are many skin illnesses that can't be dealt with as effectively as parchedness, such as skin dryness. Although it can be therapeutically treated to a certain degree, someone who is born with dry skin will always have that condition. Cannabis offers many advantages to skin treatment, such as mitigating, cancer prevention agent and soothing properties.There's no denying that marijuana is having a significant moment. Much obliged to widespread use in the medical and wellness enterprises owing to its wellbeing benefits, cannabis is currently a growing trend in the beauty world — and for great reason. As the drive for more natural, economical skin care increases skin health management products are presently touting cannabis. With the expanding trend of organic beauty items like African black soap taking the market by storm, cannabis skincare products are being seen in the structure of cannabis-infused topicals like oils, ointments, creams, balms, and lotions.Cannabis used in most skincare utilizes non-psychoactive CBD (cannabidiol) rather than THC, the psychoactive compound in maryjane, in this way making them completely lawful. Even if it does contain follow sums of THC, cannabis infusions act on a peripheral premise and do not enter the bloodstream. Therefore, it can be safely used with zero psychoactive effects on your body or the risks of bombing a medication test.

Cannabis Helps with Skin Irritation

Cannabis, when applied, topically, offer localized pain help while reducing swelling making them ideal to help with bug bites, scratches, and other skin abrasions. The application of CBD unwinds and soothes skin and can be used to treat rashes, dry skin, and more serious skin conditions like atopic dermatitis (AD), which is the most common type of dermatitis. What's more, the high concentration of polyunsaturated fatty acids present in cannabis can help to assuage the tingling and irritation related with skin inflammation. According to research from the National Eczema Association (NEA), cannabinoids tie to receptors in the skin that could decrease the indications and appearance of AD.

Cannabis Alleviates Symptoms of Psoriasis

Psoriasis is a skin disease that is characterized by itchy, painful red patches on the skin. Currently, there is no known cure for the condition. Cannabis, however, is proving to be a powerful treatment for psoriasis. According to an investigation, the cannabinoids in cannabis was discovered to hinder the buildup of dead skin cells – a direct cause of psoriasis. While more examination is needed, anecdotal evidence proposes cannabis as a potential treatment for psoriasis.

Cannabis Helps With Skin Aging

Cannabis, when applied topically, is found to slow the skin maturing process. A study uncovered that the CBD found in cannabis is a more strong antioxidant than vitamin C or E, making it viable in the treatment of wrinkles and fine lines. In addition, they additionally neutralize free radicals and keep them from damaging the collagen and elastin in your skin, keeping your skin tight and energetic in appearance. So not just does cannabis make your skin looking more young, it likewise keeps it healthier.

Cannabis Can Combat Acne

Cannabis is loaded with essential fatty acids which give hydration that is regularly discovered to be lacking in people with acne. Its antibacterial properties can help treat the bacterial contamination on the skin which is a significant contributor to acne. Cannabis skincare products are non-comedogenic, meaning it won't obstruct pores, they have calming properties, and they're rich in antioxidants. Moreover, another study indicated that CBD cannabidiol repressed and helped regulate lipid creation, helping to battle excessively oily skin. Another investigation demonstrated that the cannabinoids in cannabis can improve the appearance of skin break out because they are natural anti-inflammatories and can help to decrease the inflammation of active acne.

Cannabis Fights Bacterial Skin Infections

According to an examination, cannabis contains antimicrobial and antibacterial properties that can help in battling skin diseases. Both THC and CBD, the most popular compounds in cannabis, were found to give relief to numerous bacterial skin infections like boils, cellulitis, impetigo, and even folliculitis. Concurring to an investigation, cannabis fights against MRSA, a bacterium that causes difficult-to-treat infections since it does not respond to many anti-microbials. MSRA or Methicillin-safe Staphylococcus aureus causes diseases in different parts of the body, causing a life-threatening contamination.

Cannabis Boosts the Protective Shield

Cannabis contains vitamin A and D that contribute to the skin's natural barrier work as they stimulate cell regeneration for healthier skin. The vitamins in cannabis help to protect the skin against damage from the sun, smoke, and other ecological pollutants. Moreover, fatty acids also secure and strengthen your skin's external layer, giving you sound and more radiant skin. So far, cannabis is the single regular and non-bothering ingredient that is known to help with a number of skin afflictions. Though the use of cannabis in skincare is still fairly new, as logical examination into the therapeutic applications of cannabis proceeds, it is conceivable that even more benefits for skin will be revealed. It's no wonder that topical application of CBD skincare items is working its way into the skincare regimen of cannabis believers and skeptics alike.

Cannabis Skin Cream Recipe

Topical creams containing hemp and marijuana are a great way to improve your skin.

We've put together this recipe for a hand crafted skin treatment. Simply apply the mask to the skin for 15-20 minutes and then wash it off for healthier looking skin.

Materials

A blender

1 ripe avocado

Hemp oil

Fundamental oils, like mint or lavender (optional)

Directions

Cut up the avocado and put the pieces in the blender

Add ¼ cup of hemp oil

Add a few drops of your essential oil

Blend until mixed well

Eliminate the mixture and set aside in a bowl

Set up a large bowl of steaming hot water

Bow your head over the steam and place a towel over your head to create a facial steam bath. Hold for up to 10 minutes. (This is to open your pores so you get the maximum benefit from the cream)

Apply the mixture to your face as a mask and leave it for 15-20 minutes.

Wash off the mask and pat your skin dry with a clean towel.

Cannabis and Lavender Fizzy Bath Bombs

These are a patient favorite for relaxing after an upsetting day and easing pain as well as softening and moisturizing the skin.

Ingredients

1 Cup Baking Soda

1/2 Cup Citric Acid (found with the canning supplies)

1/2 Cup Corn Starch

1 Tablespoon Witch Hazel (found at the pharmacy)

3 Tablespoons Cannabis Coconut Oil (melted)

20 drops of Lavender

Essential Oil

5-6 drops purple food coloring

A huge mixing bowl

a strainer

latex or other gloves

2 small Dixie cups (the ones they make for bathroom dispenser)

a spoon for mixing

a cookie sheet lined with wax paper

measuring cups and spoons

Directions

In a huge blending bowl sieve together the heating soft drink corn starch and citric acid.

In a separate bowl add melted coconut oil, witch hazel and lavender oil. These will not blend together at this point yet that is OK.

Put on your gloves. Slowly add the wet fixings into the large blending bowl and begin to blend together with your gloved hands. Add a little at a time to prevent the citric acid from reacting and foaming up. In the event that it foams a little bit it will still be fine. Continue gathering and working the wet and dry ingredients into a single unit until you have a well blended blend. It will be a sodden powder. You will know when it is completely blended when the entire mixture has a uniform lavender color.

Freely measure out 1/4 Cup of your blend and place in the small Dixie cup.

Pack this tightly using a small spice jar to press it into the cup.

Transform the cup onto your wax paper lined cookie sheet. At that point if fundamental tap the bottom of the Dixie cup to release the shower bomb. Repeat this step until you've used all of your mixture and your cookie sheet has 10-11 bath bombs.

Set the treat sheet aside somewhere where these can dry and set up. Depending on your mugginess this can take 1-3 days.

After your Cannabis and Lavender Fizzy Bath Bombs have dried, store them in a resealable jar in a cool place or bundle them individually and share with your friends.

Note: If you live in a warm atmosphere or keep your home very warm you may need to store these in the ice chest as the coconut oil will melt at around 72-73 degrees F

How To Use Them:

Run yourself a warm bath. Drop in a Cannabis and Lavender Fizzy Bath Bomb. Soak in the tub for at least 20 minutes. Relax and enjoy!

Cannabis Infused Sensual Lavender Body Oil

Cannabis has had a very long standing reputation in history as a extraordinary sexual enhancer. When smoked or ingested at the right portion it increases feelings with the sentiments of touch, coaxes the flame of desire, prolongs climax, relives physical or enthusiastic torment blockages, slackens the body up, opens the psyche to new encounters, and interfaces accomplices past the physical into the realm of the soul.

Couples that get high together generally stay together as the plant serves to promote a deep cultivated bond between people. When cannabis is used in conjunction with essential oil treatment the cannabis helps to relax the body topically while the essential oils start to take hold of the faculties to help get one in the mood. This specific formula calls upon the power of Sandalwood, Rose, and Bergamot essential oils. Sandalwood is used as a base note of this body oil, giving it profundity and sensuality. This sexy essential oil is known for its aphrodisiac characteristics as it mimics the human pheromone alpha androsterole. Next we have the delicate middle note of Rose which is the heart of this mixture. Rose essential oil is very sensitive yet encompassing to the senses. It has the power to arouse an individual while invoking sentimental emotions. Then we have the wonderful light citrus scent of Bergamot adjusting out this body oil as a top note. Some of you may perceive this recognizable smell in Earl Gray tea or popular body sprays and aromas. This heavenly bunch of delicate citrus relaxes the body, reduces torment, soothes the nerves, and stimulates the production of dopamine and serotonin. In any case, no strain specific formula can be finished without a strain that compliments the scents of these luscious essential oils and their impacts. The strain Lavender is the gorgeous hybrid youngster of Super Skunk x Big Skunk Korean x Afghani Hawaiian. It has a sweet yet deep botanical bouquet with a very sensual spice fragrant undertone. The terpenes of this strain mesh so exotically with the fundamental oils of this body oil that simply breathing deeply from the glass vessel will induce and calm ones brain to a state of bliss. It isn't just the smell that is pleasing to the senses, as the impact of this strain will have the body unwinding topically. Your muscles will float away into unwinding just as your psyche is relieved into a state of delight. For maximum aphrodisiac effects, I would recommend smoking a joint or eating a consumable of the same strain before your massage meeting to procure the full spectrum of benefits this plant can give to you. Set the lights low, light candles, open the window to the sound of wind through the trees or the creek by your house, and let the experience take you somewhere you have never been previously.

Ingridents

¼ cup Sweet Almond Oil

2 grams fully cured ground Lavender (the strain or another strain with a similar terpene profile)

5 drops Sandalwood essential oil

5 drops Rose essential oil

5 drops Bergamot fundamental oil

Equipment:

1 sterilized dark colored glass jar

Twofold heater

Cheesecloth

Directions:

In a double boiler add the sweet almond oil and the ground Lavender. Turn your stove to around a 4 on the dial and let this mixture cook for 1 hour. After the time is up, strain through cheesecloth into a dark colored glass container of your decision. Let this mixture cool totally before going to the next step.

Once the carrier oil has cooled completely add in the fundamental oils of Sandalwood, Rose, and Bergamot. Delicately swirl the mixture in a circular motion until the essential oils are joined into the carrier oil. On the off chance that you need a more grounded scent, add 10 drops of each essential oil all things considered (add more carrier oil if you feel that the stronger scented body oil is too strong for sensitive skin).

You can your Sensual Lavender Body Oil immediately or you can let it "fix" for 24hrs prior to utilizing. By letting it cure, the scent of this body oil will deepen to a whole other level. In any case, if you want to use it right away, the essential oils and cannabis will still take your brain and body into another realm of relaxation and excitement. When this product is not being used store in a cool dark place and use within 2 weeks.

Appreciate! Use this body oil alone or in combination with edibles or flower for a wild sentimental evening!

Cannabis Root Salve oil

Start by making an implanted oil.

Ingredients:

Ground dried cannabis roots

coconut or olive oil

Strategy:

Spot ground dried roots in a crock-pot and cover with coconut or olive oil by an inch or two. Gently heat the blend over very low heat for 4-5 hours. Permit to cool. Strain and pour into dry sterilized amber bottles. (I like utilizing Worcestershire sauce bottles).

Ingredients:

8 oz infused oil

1 oz beeswax

nutrient E (as a preservative)

10-20 drops fundamental oil (discretionary, I like peppermint)

Method:

Place infused oils and beeswax over a double boiler and warm over low warmth until the wax melts. Mood killer the heat and add the essential oil and nutrient E. Pour into a glass container.

The consistency of the treatment can be adjusted depending on your inclinations.

Use less wax for a delicate treatment and more wax on the off chance that you want a thicker ointment.

When it cools you can make changes by warming and adding more oil or more wax until you get the consistency you need.

Cannabis Root Topical Oil

Did you know that every part of the cannabis plant is useful? Here's a recipe from my old buddy Dizledot that tells us how to remove a topical oil from the roots. It's just the thing for arthritis or muscle torment. Furthermore, you Puritans will be glad to know that it doesn't get you intoxicated, just relieves torment.

Don't Throw Those Root Balls Out!

Did you know that hemp or marijuana root is utilized to relieve muscular and bone aches, lessen swelling, ease torment, rejuvenates circulation, promotes cell growth, and empowers deep tissue mending. I try to use every bit of the plant, squander nothing is my motto! There are old plans out there dating back years and years archiving the use of roots and stems. In the event that you are like me and looking for a homeopathic use for the roots start with a topical liniment arrangement utilizing rubbing alcohol, dried and finely ground roots......

Ingredients:

1 root ball thoroughly cleaned and dried. Wash and re wash with water until all soil is removed from new roots. Make sure you have dried or dehydrated it to the point where the roots are no longer soft and pliable.

1 jug of 90% isopropyl alcohol (scouring alcohol)

Method

Grind root ball to a fine powder, open a bottle of 90% isopropyl alcohol (scouring alcohol), pour approximately 1/3 of contents into a separate container for storage.

Using a funnel with an opening appropriate to container, pour in ground material, shake well, then store in a dark place, shaking every few days, for 1-2 months.

Strain out material prior to utilizing, with a cheesecloth or coffee filter, apply liberally to affected area for pain relief, as needed.

Avocuddle Lube

Ingredients:

8 oz avocado oil, cold-pressed (or substitute with virgin coconut oil)

1/2 oz ground cannabis, decarbed (add more or less depending on your desired strength)

2 oz dried pineapple with no additives or sugar, optional*

Directions:

First you need to decarb your ground cannabis to activate the THC. Wrap the ground cannabis in foil and place in the oven at 310ºF for 10 to 18 minutes. You know it's ready when it begins smelling like a Christmas tree.

Set your sous vide water shower to 85ºC (185ºF).

Pour the avocado or coconut oil in zip seal bag and add the warm, decarbed trim. Seal the pack using the water displacement method and place into the water bath to sous vide for 4 hours to fully infuse.

After 4 hours, delicately remove pack from water bath and let cool.

Strain out the cannabis and solids with a fine mesh strainer or cheddar cloth and discard.

Keep the oil in a cool dim place.

Spiced Mango Massage Oil

Fixings:

4 oz virgin coconut oil, cold-pressed

pressed

1/2 oz ground cannabis, decarbed

1-inch piece ginger, thinly sliced

1 stick of cinnamon, broken in half

2 oz dried mango, papaya or jackfruit with no added substances or sugar

Directions:

First you need to decarb your ground cannabis to activate the THC. Wrap the ground cannabis in foil and place in the broiler at 310ºF for 10 to 18 minutes. You know it's ready when it starts possessing a scent like a Christmas tree.

Set your sous vide water bath to 85ºC (185ºF).

Pour the avocado oil, coconut oil, dried foods grown from the ground in zip seal bag and add the warm, decarbed trim. Seal the pack using the water dislodging method and place into the water shower to sous vide for 4 hours to completely implant.

After 4 hours, gently eliminate bag from water bath and let cool.

Strain out the cannabis and solids with a fine network strainer or cheese cloth and discard.

Keep the oil in a bottle in a cool dark place. Warm slightly by setting bottle in hot water before use.

CBD Oil For Skin: Usage, Advantages, Disadvantages

Cannabidiol oil or CBD oil is a skincare panacea that has been acquiring significance lately. Beauty brands like Sephora and NYX have introduced a range of CBD products, and others are quickly following suit. Beauty standards around the world have seen a drastic change recently. Porcelain white skin is no longer the marker of excellence; instead, taking consideration of it you have and still owning it is what is the issue here. You may breathe a sigh of relief, yet if you're somebody enduring from acne, Psoriasis, and other skill infirmities, it may lower your spirit. On the off chance that the tried and tested methods don't work for you, fret not! CBD oil may be the right alternative. Here's all you need to think about it.

What is CBD Oil?

Before we get into the details, let us understand what CBD oil is. As the name suggests, cannabidiol oil is a functioning fixing extricated from cannabis in a powdered form. Not at all like tetrahydrocannabinol (THC), CBD won't get you high as it does not have mind-altering properties. From the blossoms and leaves of hemp CBD is extracted, whose THC content is so low that testing equipment can rarely detect it. This non-intoxicating part is then blended with olive, coconut, or hemp oil to make it more malleable.

Is it safe to use CBD oil on skin?

It is generally safe to apply CBD oil directly to the skin as it is connected to causing any side impacts. In any case, while using CBD oil for face, lead a patch test first by applying a small amount to your skin to test if you're unfavorably susceptible. Similarly, be vigilant of the additives in your CBD item. Sometimes additives like alcohol or other oils may be the cause of your unfavorably susceptible reaction. Before you apply CBD oil on your skin, check the names to ensure that your item just contains CBD and the carrier oils.

Advantages of CBD oil

CBD oil benefits for skin are not simply restricted to saturating your face. Research suggests that CBD oil comes loaded with anti-inflammatory properties that fight skin break out and soothe skin inflammation inclined skin. In addition, CBD has the possibility to control excess sebum production and calm responsive skin.

CBD oil for Skin conditions like Psoriasis is a boon to many.

Psoriasis is an infection caused by extreme action of the immune system, which leads to frequent skin shedding. The phytocannabinoids present in CBD oil has the power to treat Psoriasis by supporting the immune system. With the assistance of CBD oil, some users have managed to kill Psoriasis forever.

CBD oil works to reduce wrinkles, additionally the visible signs of maturing. Since the compound is determined from a plant, it is stacked with cell reinforcements that counteract free-radical damage. By decreasing inflammation, CBD oil for wrinkles works its sorcery by covering fine lines, dullness, and lopsided skin tone.

Disadvantages of CBD Oil

CBD oil is by and large innocuous when taken appropriately by mouth or splashed under the tongue. However, some patients have detailed results like dry mouth, low BP, tipsiness, drowsiness, and signs of liver injury.

There isn't much information about the side-effects of CBD oil when applied straightforwardly on skin. It might be best to avoid CBD oil if you fall under the following category:

How to Use CBD Oil

On the off chance that you're pregnant or breast-feeding your infant, stay away from Cannabidiol products as they can be polluted with hurtful ingredients.

CBD items are affirmed for use in children who are two years old enough and older. A dose of 10 mg/kg daily is permittable as higher dosages are more liable to cause side effects.

Individuals with Liver diseases ideally need to use lower doses of CBD items as thought about to sound patients.

Those who have Parkinson's disease may need to cut down on cannabidiol usage owing to aggravated muscle movement and tremors.

Check out some of the best ways to use CBD oil for skin and acne:

CBD oil is highly porous. You can use it in the form of creams and balms.

In the event that you don't have any desire to apply CBD oil straightforwardly on skin, you can use it in the form of a pill. In the capsule form, the impacts of CBD oil will last for up to 8 hours.

Vaping is another way of getting the goodness of CBD into your system in a instant, viably.

It might come as a shock to you, today CBD is available in a wide assortment of food sources and drinks. Just like containers, the effect of CBD edibles endures for up to 8 hours.

Last however not least, We can consume CBD in the form of tinctures by placing Drops under the tongue for precise dose.

On the off chance that you are prone to skin break out and considering how to use CBD for acne, let us break it down to you. From the points mentioned above, the most effective way of treating acne using CBD oil is in the form of creams and balms.

How to choose CBD oil?

Now that you're recognizable with all the aspects of CBD oil, the most significant question is how to choose one? Well, here's how:

Scour through the label to ensure the product mentions "cannabidiol."

On the off chance that you're looking for a skincare CBD product, buy the ones which come in legitimate packaging so that its delicate components don't turn out to be less effective.

Pick a product that comes from a respectable organization that can offer lab results and are accessible to answer your queries.

Go for a full-spectrum CBD oil that contains a variety of cannabinoids and compounds. It may help to intensify the therapeutic benefits you receive.

On the off chance that you're not satisfied with a product, consider trying different ingredients or combinations of CBD.

What Is Hemp Oil?

Hemp seed oil is obtained from pressing the seeds of the cannabis plant (Cannabis sativa L.). Unrefined hemp seed oil is a dark greenish color with a mildly nutty aroma. Refined hemp seed oil is clear with little to no smell, but it doesn't contain as many of the skin-health benefits.

Hemp seed oil has become a very popular skincare ingredient. It's also used in cooking.

Cannabis, Hemp, and Marijuana

Understanding the contrasts among cannabis, hemp, and marijuana can be confusing on the grounds that weed and hemp all come from the same plant, Cannabis sativa. The differentiation is the variety of the plant.

Cannabis is the name of a family of plants. Hemp is an assortment inside this family, and marijuana is another assortment in the family.

Think of the sorts of tomatoes you find at the staple store, like big beefsteak tomatoes versus small Roma tomatoes. Both come from the same plant (tomato vine) yet are different varieties, and in this way, they produce diverse results if you were to cook with them. They would change in supplements, taste, texture, and more. In the case of cannabis, the varieties differ in the amount of tetrahydrocannabinol (THC) that they contain. THC is the psychoactive constituent responsible for the high that cannabis gives. Hemp by and large contains very little THC, so it has no psychoactive effects. As a result, hemp seed oil contains follow to no sums of THC. (This, in any case, is under some examination as some considers have shown that certain hemp seed oils may have detectable levels of THC. This could be the result of the oil becoming contaminated with other parts of the hemp plant during creation.) Hemp seed oil won't get you high. What's more, hemp seed oil is legal to be used and sold in skincare products.

Hemp Oil vs. CBD Oil

Hemp oil and cannabidiol (CBD) oil are also often confused with one another. Although they are acquired from the same plant, hemp oil and CBD oil are very extraordinary.

CBD is a chemical compound found in the cannabis plant (both marijuana and hemp). You may be surprised to learn that hemp seed oil is normally rich in CBD.

Hemp seed oil is comprised of a wide variety of different mixes, with CBD being just a minuscule part. CBD is found throughout the entire plant, including stalks, seeds, leaves, and flowers.

While hemp seed oil is produced by simply pressing the seeds of the hemp plant, CBD oil is created by extracting and isolating the CBD compound. This compound is then mixed with different fixings to create a CBD product. Olive oil is most often used as a base to create a CBD oil.

CBD itself does not have psychoactive impacts, however it can be formulated with THC for a product that does cause a high.1? CBD oil is frequently utilized for medicinal purposes.

Hemp-separated CBD oil is also utilized in over-the-counter skincare products, yet it's not almost as common a cosmetic fixing as hemp seed oil.

It's also important to know that hemp oil isn't the same as

marijuana oil or cannabis oil, either. Cannabis oil is extracted from the entire plant and has both CBD and THC. Cannabis oil is legitimate just in states that have legalized marijuana.

Skincare Benefits

Hemp oil is widely incorporated in many skincare products and cosmeceuticals. In fact, it's become quite a trendy ingredient. Hemp oil is not just trendy, but it can offer benefits for your skin.

Moisturizing

This is the biggest and most well-verified benefit that hemp seed oil can convey. Hemp oil is emollient and leaves the skin feeling delicate and supple.

Antioxidant Qualities

Hemp seed oil is high in antioxidant constituents: greasy acids like gamma-linolenic acid (GLA), and nutrients A, C, and E.

Antioxidant skincare products may help give your skin some protection against premature aging.2?

Anti-Inflammatory

Hemp oil contains parts that have anti-inflammatory properties, and current research suggests it might help relieve skin inflammation.3? There's more research that needs to be done here, however, to fully understand how this works on the skin.

Possible Antibacterial Qualities

Studies also recommend that hemp oil has antibacterial qualities. What effect this has on the skin, assuming any, is still being looked at. Hemp oil, CBD oil, and other cannabinoids are being studied as possible treatments for a vast array of skin conditions like acne, dermatitis, psoriasis, rosacea, and skin cancer.

Drawbacks or Side Effects

Hemp seed oil has no side effects on its own, although it's possible you may be sensitive to the ingredient.

When trying any new skincare product for the first time, be on the lookout for any signs of irritation: redness, itching, burning, or rash. If you notice any of these, stop using the offending product and give your physician a call if irritation doesn't improve after several days.

Choosing a Hemp Oil Product

Hemp oil is joined in numerous cosmetic products, from cleansers, lotions, demulcents and salves, facial items, and bath products.

Take a look at the fixing listing.

Sometimes makers will put just a small amount of hemp oil in the product, just so they can market their product as an in vogue "hemp" item. Hemp oil needn't be the first fixing, yet it shouldn't be last, all things considered.

Consider your skincare goals.

Don't simply choose a skincare item simply because it contains hemp oil. Consider what the item is planned to do and see if it adjusts with your skin's needs. For example, if your skin is dry, you'll be happier with a more emollient cream rather than a light lotion.

Look at the other fixings.

The other ingredients in a product are going to have a lot to do with how the product functions, as well. For example, if you're looking for a highly moisturizing item, one that also contains hyaluronic corrosive is a good bet. For against maturing, retinol or glycolic acid are good additions.

Examination.

All hemp oil skincare products are going to feel differently on the skin. In the event that you don't care for one, don't be shy about switching it out for another brand you may like better.

How to Use Hemp Oil for Your Skin

You may decide to swear off the locally acquired products and apply unrefined hemp seed oil directly on the skin, too.

Hemp seed oil is considered a "dry" oil. This means it absorbs rather quickly and has a non-oily feel, as far as lipid oils go.

Hemp oil is considered noncomedogenic, which means it isn't likely to clog your pores.

Some ideas for utilizing hemp seed oil:

Massage a few drops over a cleansed and saturated face, for a DIY facial serum.

Apply after bathing or showering as a body oil.

Use as a carrier oil in fragrance based treatment.

Unrefined hemp seed oil is fragile and can rapidly go rancid. To broaden its shelf life, keep your hemp oil in the fridge.

Advantages & Negatives In Marijuana In Skin

This may mean men and women getting anti-epilepsy therapeutic drugs next to CBD may request Verify A CBD products and services help you to guide assemble and maintain a sense agreeable, coupled with support totally focus in addition to the deal utilizing in frequent everyday stresses. A particular investigation established that doasage sums for procuring using CBD Gasoline pertaining to Rigidity above 1000 milligrams will cause for all intents and purposes any low affect liver-colored stomach related enzymes, yet yet the usage is probably odd rather than recommendable. When you need to discover the best CBD pieces conceivable, now ensure that they truly are in truth lab-tested. Further, medication want benzodiazepines can be obsessive and even may cause drug abuse CBD engine oil reveals promises when combat relating to each despair and furthermore nervousness, big a number of so, who take up residence simple side impacts being considering this natural procedure. Intended for programs crafted from CBD gave by hangman's rope, what's more Denver colorado does not need to need review on the executed product. It has subjected opportunities for ones legalization for the cannabis content cannabidiol (CBD) – despite the truth you still want to determine local area codes designed for legality on your area. To discover for the many perks about CBD vape gas find numerous of our maximum guide. While research and also progress for a few varieties This U.S. Diet as well as Medications Control never have affirmed using CBD discovered in servings and also refreshments. It may not be very much like commonly the non-standardised, thick CBD skin oils that have changing degrees of CBD and could are offered within wellness food shops. Artificially, CBD is undeniably involving 85 substances known as cannabinoids, which often are generally around the cannabis plant. For the reason that a student interested in cannabis CBD petroleum accessible for purchase, you could discover almost bounty of choices on brand names, product "segment, " pct CBD, tastes, amount, or anything else – any organic parcels of items may truthfully (and understandably) turned out to be overpowering. CBD petrol fails to have and even negligible records associated with THC that may potentially be a psychoactive cannabinoid and then manages the particular all around recognized marihuana high. Halter motor oil is definitely ingredient got by just chilled holding that signs of this cannabis herb (Cannabis Sativa). Found in creature investigation, THC presents debilitated generally victories throughout trimming seizures has been been proven to become a less effective anticonvulsant than CBD THC, as being a psychoactive materials, offers you plenty of unhealthy benefits, including the well-determined euphoric "huge" connected to recreational apply – that is definitely an important disincentive for those pharmaceutical administration to decide on medicines including it. His or her's skin oils keep on being total as long as they do business with a great value CO2 origin treatment, in which loans it again diminished cost

conclusions

Marijuana is like a twofold edged sword when it comes to your skin. The cancer prevention agents in marijuana seem to have an advantageous, protective effect on the skin. Marijuana likewise shows promise as a treatment for several skin conditions, including skin cancer. However, when weed is smoked, harmful byproducts can cause free radical damage to the skin and quicken signs of aging. The best ways to use marijuana for your skin are vaporizing, edibles, or topicals. When used correctly, marijuana can prompt better, more youthful-looking skin.

Made in the USA
Columbia, SC
10 September 2023